When the doctor isn't in

The challenge of taking charge of your own health

Skylar Brown

Table of Contents

*Principles of herbal medicine

*Respiratory illnesses

Chapter 1

Introduction to when the doctor isn't in

When the Doctor Isn't In is a compelling and informative book that delves deep into the world of healthcare beyond the typical doctor-patient interaction. Written by a seasoned healthcare leader, this thought-provoking book takes readers on a journey through the many facets of the healthcare industry, from insurance to hospital administration to public policy.

Drawing on real-life stories and experiences, the author sheds light on the behind-the-scenes workings of healthcare, including the challenges and obstacles faced by patients and providers alike. Readers will gain a nuanced understanding of the complexities of healthcare delivery, and will emerge with a greater appreciation for the diverse roles that healthcare professionals play in keeping our communities healthy.

This book is an essential read for anyone interested in the inner workings of the healthcare system, from patients and their families to healthcare professionals, policymakers, and anyone interested in improving healthcare outcomes for all. With its engaging storytelling and insightful analysis, When the Doctor Isn't In is a must-read for anyone looking to deepen their understanding of this critical part of our society.

Common ailments in humans

There are a wide range of common ailments that affect humans on a regular basis. Some of these common ailments include:

Common Cold: This is a viral infection that affects the upper respiratory tract. Symptoms include runny nose, sore throat, sneezing, cough, and fatigue.

Flu: This is similar to the common cold, but is caused by a different virus. Symptoms include fever, body aches, chills, and fatigue.

Headaches: There are many different types of headaches, including tension headaches, migraines, sinus headaches, and cluster headaches. They can be caused by a variety of factors, including stress, dehydration, and allergies.

Allergies: Allergies occur when the immune system overreacts to a substance that is normally harmless. Symptoms can include sneezing, itching, watery eyes, and runny nose.

Asthma: This is a chronic condition that affects the lungs. It causes inflammation and narrowing of the airways, making it difficult to breathe. Symptoms can include wheezing, coughing, and shortness of breath.

Arthritis: This is a condition that affects the joints, causing pain and stiffness. There are many different types of arthritis, including osteoarthritis, rheumatoid arthritis, and psoriatic arthritis.

Diabetes: This is a condition that affects the way the body processes glucose (sugar). There are two types of diabetes: type 1 and type 2. Symptoms can include increased thirst, frequent urination, blurred vision, and fatigue.

High Blood Pressure: This is a condition in which the force of blood against the walls of the arteries is too high. It can cause damage to the arteries and increase the risk of heart disease and stroke.

Depression: This is a mental health condition that causes feelings of sadness, hopelessness, and loss of interest in activities. It can have a significant impact on a person's quality of life.

Anxiety: This is a condition that causes excessive worry and fear. It can manifest as physical symptoms like sweating, shaking, and heart palpitations.

While these are just a few of the many common ailments humans face, it's important to seek medical attention if any symptoms persist or worsen over time.

Emergency situations

Assess the situation: The first step in dealing with a health emergency situation is to assess the situation. Is there a danger to the person or others around them? How serious is the situation?

Call for help: If the situation is serious, call for emergency medical services immediately. Provide your location, name, and a brief description of the situation.

Administer first aid: If you have first aid training, provide initial care until professional medical help arrives. This can include CPR, stopping bleeding, or giving someone medication.

Stay calm: It is important to stay calm in a health emergency situation. This will help you think clearly and make sound decisions. If you are with someone who is panicking, try to remain calm and reassure them.

Follow instructions: If you are on the phone with emergency services, follow their instructions carefully. They will provide specific guidance on what to do until medical help arrives.

Give information: Be prepared to provide information about the person's medical history, allergies, and any medication they may be taking. This will help medical professionals provide the best care possible.

Keep the person comfortable: If the person is conscious, keep them calm and comfortable. Keep them warm and reassure them that help is on the way.

Stay with them: If possible, stay with the person until medical help arrives. This can help to keep them calm and allow you to provide any necessary information to emergency services.

Home remedies

Health home remedies are a natural and effective way to treat common illnesses and ailments without having to rely on pharmaceutical drugs. These remedies are often easy to make at home with ingredients that are readily available in our kitchens and gardens, and have been used for centuries to promote healing and wellness.

Here are some popular health home remedies:

Ginger tea: Boil fresh ginger root in water to make a tea that helps relieve nausea, indigestion, and sore throat.

Honey and lemon for sore throat: Mix honey, lemon juice, and warm water and drink it to help soothe a sore throat.

Saline nasal rinse: Mix salt and warm water, and use a neti pot to flush out nasal passages to relieve sinus congestion and nasal inflammation.

Turmeric milk: Mix grated turmeric root or powder in milk and drink it before bed to relieve inflammation and improve sleep quality.

Garlic for immune health: Eat raw garlic or mix garlic paste in honey to boost the immune system and prevent cold and flu.

Apple cider vinegar for acid reflux: Mix apple cider vinegar with water and drink it before meals to relieve acid reflux symptoms.

Aloe vera gel for sunburn: Apply aloe vera gel or juice on sunburned skin to soothe the skin and reduce inflammation.

Ginger: Ginger is a natural anti-inflammatory that can help reduce pain and swelling. It's also a great digestive aid, especially for those with nausea.

Echinacea: Echinacea is often used to treat colds and flu because it helps boost the immune system. It can also help fight infections and reduce inflammation.

Lavender: Lavender has calming effects and is often used to treat anxiety and stress. It can also help with insomnia and headaches.

Chamomile: Chamomile is a natural sedative that can help with sleep and relaxation. It's also anti-inflammatory and can help with digestive issues.

Turmeric: Turmeric is known for its anti-inflammatory properties and is often used to treat arthritis and other conditions involving inflammation.

Peppermint: Peppermint can help with digestive issues, including nausea, bloating, and gas. It also has pain-relieving properties and can be used to treat headaches and muscle pain.

Milk Thistle: Milk Thistle can help support liver function and improve liver health. It's also anti-inflammatory and can help with digestive issues.

Valerian root: Valerian root is a natural sedative that can help with sleep and relaxation. It's also been used to treat anxiety and depression.

St. John's Wort: St. John's Wort is often used to treat depression and anxiety. It's also anti-inflammatory and may have other health benefits.

Garlic: Garlic is known for its immune-boosting properties and can help fight infections. It's also been shown to help reduce cholesterol and blood pressure.

Chapter 2

Understanding your body anatomy and physiology

Begin with the basics: Start with the fundamentals such as the different types of cells that make up the body and their functions.

Use visual aids: Utilize diagrams, models, and 3D visualization tools to help you understand the structures and functions of the human body.

Seek guidance from experts: Consult professionals such as physicians, anatomists, and physiologists who can guide you on how to learn human body anatomy and physiology.

Study in parts: Focus on one system at a time to avoid information overload and help you to assimilate information quickly and adequately.

Study daily: Anatomy and physiology are vast subjects. Learn continually by dedicating at least 30 minutes to 1 hour a day to study.

Read extensively: Read books, articles, and scientific journals related to anatomy and physiology to expand your knowledge.

Practice self-assessment: Test your knowledge regularly by taking quizzes and assessments to determine the areas you need to improve on.

Learn through observation: Observe the human body closely, especially during dissections, to understand its anatomical features better.

CPR (cardiopulmonary resuscitation)

Bandaging cuts and wounds

Treating burns by cooling the affected area and covering it with a sterile dressing

Administering pain relief medication

Treating insect bites and stings

Giving an epinephrine injection for severe allergic reactions

Applying cold compresses or ice packs for injuries that cause swelling or inflammation

Treating nosebleeds by tilting the head forward and pinching the nostrils closed

Providing treatment for shock, such as lying down and elevating the feet

Administering an asthma inhaler for breathing difficulties.

Treating allergies

Identify the allergen: If you know what's causing your allergy, try to avoid it. If it's not clear what's causing your symptoms, see an allergist for a skin or blood test.

Medications: Antihistamines, decongestants, and steroid nasal sprays can help reduce allergy symptoms. Over-the-counter or prescription-strength options are available.

Allergy shots: If medications aren't working or you're experiencing severe symptoms, immunotherapy (allergy shots) may help.

Nasal irrigation: This involves rinsing your nasal passages with a saltwater solution.

Lifestyle changes: Reduce exposure to allergens by keeping windows closed, washing bedding in hot water weekly, and showering after spending time outdoors.

Consult a doctor: If your symptoms persist, worsen or interfere with your normal daily activities, consult with a doctor for guidance.

Digestive disorder

Digestive disorder is a medical condition that affects the digestive system that includes the esophagus, stomach, pancreas, liver, gallbladder, small and large intestines. These disorders can range from simple problems like indigestion and constipation to more complex conditions like inflammatory bowel disease, irritable bowel syndrome, celiac disease, and gastroesophageal reflux disease. These disorders can cause discomfort, pain, bloating, diarrhea, and other symptoms that can affect the quality of life of the patient. They can be caused by various factors like poor diet, stress, infections, genetics, and structural abnormalities. Treatment options depend on the type and severity of the condition and may include medication, surgery, lifestyle changes, and dietary modifications.

Consult with a doctor to determine the cause of the digestive disorder and follow their prescribed treatment plan.

Avoid trigger foods that exacerbate symptoms, such as high-fat or spicy dishes.

Eat smaller and more frequent meals to prevent overloading the digestive system.

Stay hydrated by drinking plenty of water throughout the day.

Reduce stress through exercise, meditation, or other relaxation techniques.

Incorporate probiotics and prebiotics into your diet to help promote healthy gut flora.

Try natural remedies like ginger,

peppermint, or chamomile to help alleviate symptoms.

Avoid smoking and excessive alcohol consumption, as they can irritate the digestive system.

Remember, it is always best to consult with a healthcare provider before starting any new treatment or making significant changes to your diet.

Understanding nutrients

Understanding human nutrients involves knowing the different types of nutrients that the human body needs to function properly, their sources, and their roles in the body. The following are the types of nutrients that the body needs:

Carbohydrates: Carbohydrates are the main source of energy for the body. They are found in foods such as grains, fruits, and vegetables.

Proteins: Proteins are essential for the growth and repair of the body's tissues. They are found in foods such as meat, fish, eggs, and soy.

Fats: Fats provide energy, insulation, and protection for the body's organs. They are found in foods such as oils, nuts, seeds, and fatty fish.

Vitamins: Vitamins are essential for the normal functioning of the body. They are found in foods such as fruits, vegetables, and fortified foods.

Minerals: Minerals are important for the proper functioning of the body's systems. They are found in foods such as dairy products, green leafy vegetables, and meat.

By understanding these different nutrients, their functions in the body, and the foods that provide them, one can ensure that their body receives the nutrients it needs for optimal health.

Chapter 3

Medical conditions on different chronic diseases

Diabetes: a chronic disease characterized by high blood sugar levels due to insufficient insulin production or resistance in the body. It can lead to complications such as cardiovascular disease, kidney damage, nerve damage, and blindness.

Hypertension: also known as high blood pressure, it is a chronic medical condition characterized by increased pressure in the arteries. This can cause damage to the heart, kidneys, brain, and other organs and is a major risk factor for heart disease, stroke, and kidney failure.

Arthritis: a chronic disease that affects the joints and surrounding tissues, causing pain, stiffness, and swelling. It can be caused by various factors, including age, genetics, and autoimmune disorders.

Chronic Obstructive Pulmonary Disease (COPD): a group of lung diseases including emphysema and chronic bronchitis that cause breathing difficulties due to damage to the lungs over time. It is mainly caused by smoking and can lead to chronic respiratory failure.

Asthma: a chronic inflammatory disease that affects the airways in the lungs, causing wheezing, shortness of breath, and chest tightness. It can be triggered by allergens or irritants in the environment and can be managed through medication and lifestyle changes.

Chronic kidney disease: a condition that occurs when the kidneys are not functioning properly, leading to a buildup of waste in the body. It can be caused by diabetes, hypertension, and other factors and can progress over time to end-stage renal disease, requiring dialysis or a kidney transplant.

Heart disease: a broad term for different conditions that affect the heart, including coronary artery disease, heart failure, and arrhythmias. It is a leading cause of death worldwide and can be caused by various factors such as smoking, high blood pressure, and diabetes.

Cancer: a group of diseases characterized by the uncontrolled growth and spread of abnormal cells. It can affect any part of the body and has many different types and subtypes, each with its unique symptoms, treatments, and prognoses.

Medical test of health disorders

There are several medical tests that can be conducted to diagnose various health disorders. A few examples include:

Blood tests: These tests are used to check for various medical conditions by analyzing blood samples. Examples include complete blood count (CBC), blood glucose levels, cholesterol levels, and thyroid function tests.

Imaging tests: These tests are used to visualize internal tissues and organs to diagnose medical conditions. Examples include X-rays, CT scans, MRI scans, and ultrasounds.

Electrocardiogram (ECG): This test records the electrical activity of the heart to help diagnose heart conditions such as arrhythmia, heart attack, or heart failure.

Biopsy: A tissue or cell sample is taken and examined under a microscope to diagnose various conditions, including cancer.

Pulmonary function tests: These tests measure how well the lungs are functioning and are used to diagnose conditions such as asthma, chronic obstructive pulmonary disease (COPD), and emphysema.

Endoscopy: This test involves a flexible tube with a camera and light that is inserted into the body to examine organs such as the stomach, intestines, or lungs.

Allergy tests: These tests are used to identify allergens that may be causing an allergic reaction.

Urine tests: These tests are used to detect conditions such as urinary tract infections, kidney disease, or diabetes by analyzing urine samples.

Diagnostic procedures

Diagnostic procedure is the series of tests, evaluations, and investigations used by healthcare professionals to determine the cause, nature, and severity of a patient's health issue or disease. It can include physical examination, laboratory tests, imaging techniques, medical history review, and other medical procedures to ascertain the patient's condition. The diagnostic procedure generally involves a systematic approach that enables the identification of the patient's health problems and the development of effective treatment plans. The aim of diagnostic procedures is to obtain an accurate diagnosis that can guide the medical team in developing a tailored treatment strategy for the patient.

Preventive medicine

Preventive medicines, also known as prophylactic medicines or preventative medications, are drugs intended to prevent the occurrence or progression of a disease or condition. These medications may be recommended for individuals who have a high risk or vulnerability to a particular disease or condition.

Some examples of preventive medicines include:

Vaccines: These are medications that aim to prevent disease by stimulating the body's natural immune response.

Antibiotics: These medicines are used to prevent bacterial infections.

Statins: These medications are used to lower cholesterol and prevent heart disease.

Aspirin: This medication is often used to prevent heart attacks and strokes.

Contraceptives: These medications are used to prevent unwanted pregnancies.

Pre-exposure prophylaxis (PrEP): This medication is used to prevent the transmission of HIV.

Antimalarials: These medications are used to prevent and treat malaria.

Chemoprevention drugs: These medications are used to prevent the development of cancer or to prevent its recurrence in individuals who have had cancer in the past.

Fluoride supplements: These medications are used to prevent tooth decay.

Maintaining good health

Eat a balanced and nutritious diet: Include plenty of fruits, vegetables, whole grains, lean proteins, and healthy fats in your diet.

Exercise regularly: Engage in physical activities that you enjoy, such as running, swimming, dancing, or walking, for at least 30 minutes a day.

Get enough sleep: Aim for 7-8 hours of sleep every night to help your body recuperate and recover.

Manage stress: Practice stress-relieving activities such as meditation, yoga, or deep breathing to reduce the chances of developing chronic illnesses.

Stay hydrated: Make sure you drink plenty of water to keep your body hydrated and maintain optimal body functions.

Avoid harmful substances: Quit smoking, limit your alcohol intake, and stay away from drugs to reduce your risk of developing addiction and harmful health conditions.

Regular checkups: Get regular health screenings and checkups, including dental and vision examinations, to detect any health issues early on.

Maintain social connections: Connect with friends and family members, join community events, and participate in social activities to promote social well-being and mental health.

Maintain personal hygiene: Practice good personal hygiene, such as washing hands regularly, brushing teeth twice a day, and showering regularly, to prevent the spread of germs.

Stay informed: Stay informed about health issues and take an active role in your healthcare by regularly reading about health topics and discussing any concerns with a healthcare professional.

Chapter 4

Coping with common health issues

Headaches: Rest, relax, and avoid triggers like loud noise or strong smells. Consider natural remedies like peppermint oil or ginger tea.

Colds and Flu: Rest, stay hydrated, and take over-the-counter medication like pain relievers, decongestants, or cough suppressants. Consider natural remedies like echinacea, zinc lozenges, or elderberry syrup.

Back Pain: Rest, apply ice or heat, and take over-the-counter pain medication like acetaminophen, ibuprofen, or naproxen. Consider natural remedies like yoga, massage, or acupuncture.

Anxiety and Depression: Seek professional help, therapy, or medication. Maintain a healthy lifestyle by exercising regularly, eating a balanced diet, and getting enough sleep.

Digestive Issues: Avoid trigger foods, stay hydrated, and take over-the-counter medication like antacids, laxatives, or probiotics. Consider natural remedies like peppermint tea, ginger, or chamomile tea.

Remember, always consult with your doctor or healthcare provider to get the most appropriate and effective treatment for your individual health issue.

Self help strategies on health

Eat a balanced and wholesome diet: Eating a well-balanced diet rich in nutrients and vitamins is essential in maintaining good health. Include fruits, vegetables, lean proteins, whole grains, and healthy fats in your diet.

Stay hydrated: Drinking plenty of water throughout the day helps flush out toxins from your body and keeps your system functioning properly.

Exercise regularly: Regular exercise helps improve overall health, boosts immunity, and reduces the risk of chronic diseases. It can also help with weight management, elevate mood, and reduce stress.

Get enough sleep: Getting enough sleep is crucial for maintaining good health. It helps you feel refreshed, energized, and ready to tackle the day.

Reduce stress: Chronic stress can lead to a number of health issues, including depression, anxiety, heart disease, and diabetes. Practice relaxation techniques like meditation, yoga, or deep breathing exercises to manage stress.

Avoid harmful habits: Avoid smoking, excessive alcohol consumption, and drug abuse. These habits can have serious negative impacts on your health.

Take breaks and practice self-care: Taking breaks, engaging in hobbies and activities that you enjoy, and practicing self-care can help reduce stress and help you feel more balanced.

Stay connected: Maintaining social connections is important for overall health and well-being. Spending time with loved ones, participating in group activities, and making new friends are all ways to stay connected.

Monitor your health: Regular monitoring of blood pressure, cholesterol, blood sugar, and other key health indicators can help identify potential health issues early and allow for timely intervention.

Seek professional help when needed: Don't hesitate to seek professional help when needed. A physician, therapist, or other medical professional can provide expert guidance on how to maintain good health and manage any health concerns that arise.

Chronic pain

Chronic pain is a medical condition that is defined as pain that persists for more than three months. It is often the result of an injury, illness, or disease, and it can be severe enough to interfere with a person's daily activities and quality of life. Chronic pain is a complex condition that requires a multidisciplinary approach to management, including medication, physical therapy, and psychological counseling.

There are many different types of chronic pain, including neuropathic pain, which is caused by damage to the nerves; cancer pain, which is caused by a tumor or cancer treatment; and musculoskeletal pain, which is caused by damage to the bones, joints, or muscles. Chronic pain may also be associated with other conditions, such as depression, anxiety, and sleep disturbances.

Chronic pain management is a complex process that requires a collaborative effort among healthcare providers, the patient, and their support network. Treatment approaches may include medication, physical therapy, occupational therapy, acupuncture, biofeedback, and counseling. Pain management may also include lifestyle changes such as weight loss, smoking cessation, and stress reduction.

It is important to seek medical assistance for chronic pain as soon as possible, as untreated pain can lead to long-term complications and disability. In some cases, chronic pain can be completely relieved, but in other cases, it can only be managed. However, with proper care and management, people with chronic pain can lead full and productive lives.

Causes of pain

There are numerous causes of pain in human health, some of which include:

Injury: Pain can result from various types of injuries, such as fractures, strains, sprains, and bruises.

Inflammation: Inflammation can cause pain due to the release of chemicals that can stimulate nerve endings.

Infection: Infections in the body can lead to pain as the immune system responds to the presence of the invading pathogens.

Chronic diseases: Diseases such as arthritis, fibromyalgia, and multiple sclerosis can cause chronic pain due to ongoing issues in the body.

Nerve damage: Damage to nerves can cause pain as the affected nerves send incorrect or excessive signals to the brain.

Post-surgery: Post-operative pain is common, especially after invasive procedures.

Age-related changes: As the body ages, changes in the musculoskeletal system can result in painful conditions such as osteoarthritis.

Cancer: Pain can be a symptom of cancer, especially as the disease progresses.

Psychological factors: Emotional stress and mental health conditions can contribute to pain in the body.

Genetic predisposition: Some individuals may have a genetic predisposition to certain types of pain, such as migraines.

Managing pain and medication

Identify the type of pain: Pain can have different causes, such as injury, illness, diseases, or chronic conditions. Knowing the underlying cause helps in determining the appropriate treatment.

Consult a doctor: Pain management should always involve consulting with a healthcare professional. A doctor will review the patient's medical history, conduct a physical exam, and recommend appropriate medical interventions, including medications.

Follow the prescribed medication: Medications prescribed to manage pain should be taken according to the doctor's instructions. Patients should ask their doctors about any potential side effects and the right dosage.

Use alternative treatments: Apart from medication, there are other treatments to manage pain, such as physical therapy, massage, acupuncture, and cognitive-behavioral therapy. Patients can discuss with their healthcare professionals for more information on these treatments.

Monitor for severe side effects: Some pain medications can cause severe side effects such as addiction, respiratory depression, and gastrointestinal issues. Patients should be aware of any signs of side effects and contact their healthcare professionals immediately.

Take measures to prevent pain: Making lifestyle changes like eating a healthy diet, regular exercise, getting enough sleep, and avoiding triggers that cause pain can help manage pain in the long-term.

Consider long-term pain management options: If pain is chronic, other treatments like nerve blocks, implanted devices, and surgery may be necessary. Patients should discuss with their doctors about these options.

Cardiovascular issues

Cardiovascular issues are a group of medical conditions that affect the heart and blood vessels. These conditions range from mild to severe and can include high blood pressure, coronary artery disease, heart attack, stroke, arrhythmias, heart failure, and peripheral artery disease.

High blood pressure is a common cardiovascular issue that can lead to other health problems. Blood pressure measures the force of blood against the walls of the arteries as the heart pumps it through the body. Over time, high blood pressure can damage the organs and increase the risk of heart attack, stroke, and other complications.

Coronary artery disease occurs when the arteries that supply blood to the heart become narrow or blocked due to plaque buildup. This can cause angina, which is chest pain or discomfort, as well as heart attack if the artery becomes completely blocked.

A heart attack occurs when blood flow to a section of the heart muscle is blocked, leading to damage or death of the muscle tissue. The symptoms of a heart attack include chest pain or discomfort, shortness of breath, and pain in the arms, neck, jaw, or back.

Stroke is a serious cardiovascular issue that occurs when a blood vessel in the brain is blocked or bursts, leading to damage or death of brain cells. Symptoms of stroke include sudden weakness or numbness on one side of the body, trouble speaking, difficulty seeing or walking, and severe headache.

Arrhythmias are abnormal heart rhythms that can cause palpitations, dizziness, fainting, or even sudden death. Heart failure occurs when the heart is unable to pump enough blood to meet the body's needs, leading to fatigue, shortness of breath, and fluid buildup in the lungs or other parts of the body.

Peripheral artery disease occurs when the arteries that supply blood to the arms or legs become narrow or blocked. This can cause pain or numbness in the affected limb, poor wound healing, or even gangrene if left untreated.

Preventing or managing cardiovascular issues often involves making lifestyle changes such as maintaining a healthy weight, eating a balanced diet, exercising regularly, quitting smoking, and managing stress. Medications, procedures, and surgery may also be used to treat cardiovascular issues depending on the severity of the condition. It is important to seek medical attention if you experience symptoms of a cardiovascular issue to prevent complications and improve treatment outcomes.

Chapter 5

A principle of natural healing

The principle of natural healing suggests that the human body has an innate ability to heal itself when provided with the right conditions, including a healthy diet, physical activity, social connections, emotional balance, and spiritual well-being. Rather than relying solely on medication, surgeries, or invasive procedures, natural healing emphasizes the restoration of the body's natural balance and the stimulation of the body's own healing processes. It focuses on treating the root cause of the disease rather than just suppressing the symptoms, thereby promoting long-term health and well-being.

Natural healing considers various factors that affect health, including the environment, lifestyle, and genetics. It recognizes that each individual is unique, and hence, requires personalized care that addresses their specific needs. The approach of natural healing is holistic, meaning it considers the whole person, including their body, mind, and spirit.

Some of the techniques used in natural healing include herbal medicine, acupuncture, meditation, massage therapy, hydrotherapy, and nutritional therapy. The effectiveness of these methods is supported by scientific research and backed by traditional knowledge.

In conclusion, natural healing emphasizes the importance of prevention and self-care during the healing process. It recognizes the body's ability to heal itself, and hence focuses on creating conditions that support and enhance this process. It is a non-invasive, gentle, and effective path to natural health and ultimate well-being.

Components of natural healing

Proper Nutrition: Consuming a balanced diet of whole and natural foods, rich in nutrients, vitamins and minerals, is an essential aspect of natural healing.

Adequate Hydration: Adequate water consumption plays a vital role in flushing out toxins from the body, maintaining the body's pH balance, and aiding in the absorption of essential nutrients.

Exercise: Regular exercise helps improve circulation and oxygen supply throughout the body, strengthening the immune system and reducing stress levels.

Sleep: Getting proper rest and sleep at night is essential for the body to repair, rejuvenate, and regenerate.

Stress management: Managing stress through practices such as meditation, deep breathing exercises, and mindfulness can reduce the risk of chronic illness, digestive problems and boost overall well-being.

Natural Remedies: Natural remedies such as herbs, essential oils, and homeopathic remedies can be effective in treating various problems like headaches, insomnia, digestive problems, etc.

Massage Therapy: Regular massage therapy treatments help improve circulation, reduce pain, stress, and tension.

Mind-body connection: The natural healing process involves acknowledging the connection between the mind and the body, and taking care of both is crucial for overall health and well-being.

Spiritual Healing: Spiritual practices such as prayer, meditation, and yoga can provide emotional and psychological support, connection, and guidance for natural healing.

Traditional healing practices: Traditional healing practices such as acupuncture, herbal medicine, and Ayurveda can be effective in treating various health issues and promoting natural healing.

Using natural health treatment

Research: Read up on the natural health treatment you are interested in and understand its benefits and risks.

Consider your health condition: Consult a healthcare professional to determine if natural health treatments are suitable for your condition.

Choose natural remedies: Natural health treatments include herbal supplements, essential oils, and other natural-based treatments.

Adhere to dosage guidelines: Follow the recommended dosage guidelines for any natural health treatment you use.

Monitor your health: Watch for any changes in your health while using natural health treatments and report any concerning symptoms to your healthcare provider.

Principles of herbal medicines

Holistic Approach: Herbal medicines focus on treating the root cause of the condition by addressing the mind, body, and soul of the individual.

Individualized Approach: Herbal medicines are designed to suit the specific needs of the individual and take into account factors such as age, gender, medical history, and lifestyle habits.

Natural Healing: Herbal medicines are derived from plants and natural sources, and therefore do not have any synthetic additives or chemicals. They work in harmony with the body to promote healing and wellness.

Prevention and Maintenance: Herbal medicines are designed to not only treat symptoms, but also prevent conditions from occurring, and maintain overall health and well-being.

Harmlessness: Herbal medicines are generally safe, non-toxic and have fewer side effects compared to synthetic drugs if used appropriately.

Scientifically Proven: Herbal medicines are grounded in science and research, and are constantly being studied for their efficacy, safety and therapeutic value.

Integrative Approach: Herbal medicines can be used in conjunction with conventional medicine to reinforce, complement and enhance treatment outcomes.

Social and Cultural Acceptance: Herbal medicines have been used in traditional medicine for centuries and in many cultures have a strong history of use and acceptance.

Complementary Treatment: Herbal medicines are intended to complement and not replace conventional medicine, serving as an alternative option for those seeking more natural ways of healing.

Sustainable and Eco-Friendly: Herbal medicines are environmentally sustainable and play a key role in protecting our natural resources, thus promoting a healthier planet.

Respiratory illnesses

Respiratory illnesses refer to a group of diseases that affect the respiratory system, including the lungs, bronchi, trachea, and nasal passages. These can be caused by viral or bacterial infections, allergies, irritants, or other factors.

Some common respiratory illnesses include:

Asthma

Bronchitis

Chronic obstructive pulmonary disease (COPD)

Influenza (flu)

Pneumonia

Tuberculosis (TB)

Symptoms of respiratory illnesses vary depending on the specific condition, but may include coughing, wheezing, shortness of breath, chest pain, fever, and fatigue. Treatment options also vary depending on the condition, but may include medication, rest, and lifestyle changes. In some cases, more severe respiratory illnesses may require hospitalization or other medical interventions.

www.ingramcontent.com/pod-product-compliance
Lightning Source LLC
Chambersburg PA
CBHW061557250726

48657CB00021B/2060